Small Space Fitness and Nutrition

Urban Wellness Solutions

Table of Contents

Chapter 1. Introduction

Welcome to a Special Report perfectly curated for the urban dweller - "Small Space Fitness and Nutrition: Urban Wellness Solutions". As city spaces shrink and life pace quickens, it's crucial to carve out our personal oasis of health and wellbeing. This comprehensive report gleefully ushers you into the world of compact exercise regimes, nutrition hacks, and wellness techniques tailored for limited spaces. Prepare to transform your tiny condo or bustling studio apartment into a vibrant hub for fitness! Featuring expert advice, actionable tips, and innovative ideas, our report is a treasure trove designed to inspire, motivate, and guide you to achieve and maintain a dynamic, healthy lifestyle in the heart of the city. This is your golden ticket to push boundaries – only you don't need a sprawling backyard or a five-bed mansion to do it. The city is your oyster; it's time to cultivate your pearl of wellness! Dive in to unravel the countless possibilities of urban wellness hidden in your small space.

Chapter 2. Unleashing the Power of Small Spaces for Fitness

The often-overlooked beauty about fitness is it can be achieved anywhere. It doesn't require a grand, luxurious space. As an urban dweller, you can harness the versatility of fitness and transform your small space into an influential player in your quest towards better wellness. Let's delve deeper.

2.1. Understanding the Space: Limitations and Possibilities

Urban living is all about making the most of what you have, and this rings incredibly true when it comes to optimizing your living space for fitness. Here, your first step is to evaluate your current situation. Understand the practical constraints and potential offerings of your space. Keep an eye out for areas that could serve dual, or even multiple, purposes. The living room, the bedroom, or even the kitchen can convert into mini workout arenas in a matter of seconds.

2.2. Design Your Fitness Corner

Even within the smallest quarters, it's advisable to designate a specific region for your workouts. This sends a clear signal to your brain that this space means 'business', thereby mentally preparing you for the workout session. This 'fitness corner' can be as simple as a yoga mat's worth of floor space with a small shelf for your workout essentials. Eliminate clutter to make your workout area as inviting as possible.

2.3. Equipment Choices for Small Spaces

When furnishing your compact fitness corner, consider versatile equipment that can cater to different fitness regimes and require minimal storage space. Resistance bands, adjustable dumbbells, yoga mats, balance balls, and kettlebells are a few essential, space-saving suggestions. Remember, you don't need a full gym setup to stay fit.

2.4. Practicing Bodyweight Exercises and Calisthenics

Without needing any equipment, bodyweight exercises and calisthenics are ideal for building strength, endurance, and flexibility. These exercises are practical for small spaces and can be modified to suit different difficulty levels. They can range from simple movements such as squats, pushups, lunges, or jumping jacks, to more advanced exercises like burpees, pistol squats, and handstands.

2.5. Embracing Yoga and Pilates

Yoga and Pilates are terrific disciplines that require minimal space and still offer comprehensive full-body workouts. With a wide range of online lessons available – from calming Yin Yoga to dynamic Vinyasa flows or core-strengthening Pilates – you can explore various techniques right in your living room.

2.6. High-Intensity Interval Training (HIIT)

If you're on a tight schedule, HIIT workouts can be your best friend. As incredibly efficient calorie-burning sessions, HIIT exercises require less time while still radically improving your cardiovascular fitness and muscular strength. The best part is that HIIT can be tailored for small spaces – basic sprinting on the spot, jump squats, burpees, or high knees are just a few examples.

2.7. Safe Exercise Practices in Limited Spaces

While exercising in constrained spaces, it is important to exercise safely. Avoid vigorous movements in areas with fragile or sharp objects. Always ensure there's sufficient headroom for overhead exercises. Lastly, always warm up before, and cool down after exercises to reduce the risk of injuries.

2.8. Using Technology for Learning and Inspiration

Leverage digital fitness platforms and apps offering guided workouts that suit your particular space limitations. YouTube, Fitness+ by Apple, Peloton, and Fitbod are some examples of platforms providing wide-ranging options for home workouts.

2.9. A Community Approach to Fitness

Without the luxury of a backyard or nearby open space for outdoor workouts, a community approach towards fitness can work wonders. Participating in neighborhood health challenges, joining online workout classes, or even organizing building-wide fitness initiatives can amplify your health ambitions and enhance community spirit.

In essence, small space fitness is all about creativity, adaptability, and resolve. It's about realizing that the scope and degree of your fitness journey aren't dictated by physical dimensions alone. Engage these approaches, and you will find yourself successfully navigating through the challenges of small space fitness.

Chapter 3. Strategically Squeezing Exercise into Your Urban Lifestyle

Living in an urban environment brings a unique set of challenges for healthy living, especially when it comes to incorporating regular physical activities into routines crammed with work, travel, and social obligations. Fortunately, innovative and strategic ways can be employed to incorporate exercise into your life, without requiring large spaces or sacrificing precious time.

3.1. Embrace a Fitness Mindset

The first step towards integrating fitness into your city life is adopting a fitness mindset. This involves recognizing any opportunity as a chance to stay active. For instance, take the stairs instead of the elevator, or walk to run errands instead of driving. Incorporate movement into your daily tasks; doing light stretches while watching television or listening to a webinar means you're not resigned to a sedentary lifestyle.

Every bit of physical activity, no matter how small it seems, contributes to your overall fitness levels and general health. It is all about making the most of what you have, no matter how limited it seems.

3.2. Soak in the Benefits of Compact Workouts

High-intensity interval training (HIIT) offers the perfect solution for individuals confined by limited spaces or time. These are quick, intensive workouts usually lasting between 10 to 30 minutes. They involve short bursts of high-energy exercises, interspersed with brief periods of recovery. Popular workout forms include burpees, squat jumps, jumping jacks, or even stair climbing.

```
| Exercise          | Description |
|------------------|------------|
| Burpees           | Full body exercise involving a
series of squats, jumps, and push-ups. |
| Jumping jacks     | Classic cardio exercise, involving
jumping with wide arm and leg spreads. |
| Squat jumps       | Energizing exercise involving a
squat followed by a jump. |
| Stair climbing   | Great for cardiovascular health, it
involves climbing up and down stairs. |
```

```
Adding a HIIT routine to your day not only strengthens
and tones your muscles, but also boosts your metabolism
and enhances calorie-burning long after the workout.
Plus, you can do it right in your living room within a
small 2x2 meter space!
```

3.3. Blend Wellness with Work

The 'sit-stand desk' is an increasingly popular office wellness trend designed to combat the perils of a sedentary work life. By providing the flexibility to switch between sitting and standing positions, this innovative desk style promotes movement and prevents the health risks associated with prolonged sitting. Completing tasks while standing helps burn more calories, improves posture, and aids in better concentration.

In addition to the desk, consider incorporating desk-based exercise equipment like under-desk cycles or treadmill desks. These tools foster an active work environment and help you stay fit while juggling your work commitments.

3.4. The Wonders of Urban Outdoor Workouts

Cities provide several outdoor fitness opportunities - it's all about perspective. Parks offer a green oasis amidst the urban jungle for running, yoga, tai chi, or free-hand exercises. Many city parks are installed with open-air fitness equipment as well, allowing you to get a complete workout while soaking up the vitamin D.

Alternatively, consider joining older neighborhood residents in their morning or evening walk routes. Apart from the fitness aspect, neighborhood walks also offer an excellent opportunity for social interaction.

3.5. Incorporating Digital Fitness

The digital era offers a plethora of online fitness resources that cater to urban dwellers with limited spaces, from yoga and pilates to strength training and dance workouts. Fitness apps and YouTube channels provide a wide variety of at-home workout routines for different fitness levels and interests. These platforms allow you to transform any corner of your home or office into a personal fitness studio.

Remember, the key is consistency. It might seem challenging initially, but persistence will pay off in terms of improved health, fitness, and overall wellbeing. Small steps can make a big difference in enhancing your urban lifestyle. Embrace the constraints of city living and turn them into your advantage, because you are not confined by your circumstances, you're only limited by your mindset and creativity.

Chapter 4. Innovation in Compact Exercise Equipment

Innovation in compact fitness equipment has seen a drastic surge, notably due to the increasing necessity of indoor fitness regimes compatible with small living spaces. Conventional fitness machinery, with their hefty frames and limited adaptability, often fail to provide an ideal solution for urban dwellers. So, the industry has pumped up its innovation game, introducing equipment that not only saves square footage but is also as efficient as, if not more than, their traditional counterparts.

4.1. The Rise of Compactness in Fitness

The trend of compact fitness equipment has risen in parallel to the growth of micro-apartments, increased urbanization, and a higher concentration of people living in constricted city spaces. According to the American College of Sports Medicine, small-space dwelling is one of the key drivers of exercise equipment innovation. People are becoming more inclined towards products that complement their living standards by efficiently utilizing available space – giving rise to portable, stowable, and multifunctional fitness gear.

4.2. Portable Equipment Boosting Convenience

When it comes to portable exercise equipment, there's a plethora of innovations. For instance, there are jump ropes with adjustable weights, collapsible foam rollers, and foldable yoga mats — everything in this category can easily be packed and used anywhere.

Resistance bands, too, have made their mark in this category. They are lightweight and easily manipulated to cater to a variety of muscle-targeting workouts, from arms and legs to the core. Moreover, there are different resistance levels available, from light to heavy, allowing you to steadily progress.

4.3. Stowable Solutions - Space Savers

Stowable workout equipment is the holy grail for cramped studio apartments. In this sector, we have treadmills that fold vertically, thus becoming easily storable against the wall or under the bed. Similarly, compact elliptical machines comfortably fit under the desk, allowing a workout while you work.

A sublime example of stowable and portable equipment combo is TRX (Total Resistance Exercises) equipment, which includes suspension trainers. These workout tools can be attached to any secure hook and then easily stowed away after your workout, providing a diverse range of strength-based exercises.

A rising star in this category is the 'Mirror' - a smart workout system that doubles as a full-length mirror when not in use. Equipped with personalised training regimes, this interactive piece of technology has revolutionized home workouts.

4.4. Multipurpose Tools - More Bang for Your Bucks

The value of multipurpose tools is colossal, primarily for those who cannot afford an abundance of gear due to space, price, or both. Adjustable dumbbells, kettlebell/dumbbell hybrids and convertible exercise benches are some invincible stars under this category.

Adjustable dumbbells allow you to modify the weight according to your needs by simply adding or removing weight plates. The kettlebell/dumbbell hybrid serves as a kettlebell for swinging movements and integrated grip handles double it as a standard dumbbell. Convertible benches, on the other hand, are multifunctional, offering a full-bodied, varied workout.

4.5. Smart Equipment – Technology Meets Fitness

Smart fitness equipment embeds technology into your workout regime, making it more interactive and personalised. Leading the pack is the 'Peloton Bike.' Integrated with live and on-demand classes led by professional trainers, this compact bike brings the immersive group class experience into the heart of your home.

In the same vein is the high-intensity interval training equipment 'Bowflex Max Trainer.' The compact design gym-grade machine uses AI to adjust workout intensity based on individual pacing. It learns and customises itself to provide the most effective workout possible.

4.6. Eco-Friendly Innovations

Awareness of environmental sustainability is seeping into fitness equipment too. An example is the 'EcoMill,' a non-motorised treadmill, which generates its own power as you run on it. Similarly, 'SportsArt' has launched the 'VERDE,' the first energy-producing treadmill, which turns the calories you burn into usable electricity.

The realm of eco-friendly equipment is expanding with the introduction of mats made of sustainable, recyclable materials and water-powered rowing machines.

Modern compact fitness equipment is a testament to how innovation and convenience can go hand in hand. By bridging the gap between spatial constraints and lifestyle necessities, this array of new-age tools is fostering the concept of urban wellness with a compact spin. After all, when it comes to cultivating fitness in small living areas, less can indeed be more.

Chapter 5. Nutrition Masterplan for the Urban Dweller

In an urban milieu where every minute counts, eating nutritiously can be a challenge. Quick fixes and takeaway meals often rule the roost. However, a conscious shift towards healthier diets, scheduled meals, and balanced nutrition can work wonders in keeping fit, energetic, and productive. And yes, this is entirely possible even within the confines of a bustling city life.

5.1. Essential Nutrients for the Urban Dweller

The first step to creating your nutrition masterplan is understanding the types of nutrients your body needs. These fall into two categories: macronutrients and micronutrients.

Macronutrients include proteins, carbohydrates, and fats, the heart of any meal, supplying the body with energy (calories) and critical metabolic substances.

Micronutrients, much needed but in smaller amounts, include vitamins and minerals. They are vital for a robust immune system, energy production, blood clotting, and myriad other functions.

Let's cruise through each of these nutrients, looking at their importance, sources, and ideal intake.

1. Protein Protein builds, repairs, and maintains bodily tissues like muscles, skin, and hair. It's also vital in creating enzymes and hormones. While animal-based foods are high in protein,

vegetarians can consume lentils, chickpeas, and quinoa for their daily dose.

2. Carbohydrates Carbohydrates are body's primary source of energy. Whole grains, fruits, and legumes offer good amounts. Remember to limit refined carbohydrates found in sugary drinks and packaged food.

3. Fats Not all fats are bad! Certain fats, like mono and polyunsaturated fats, are essential for heart and brain health. Avocados, fish, and nuts are great sources. However, limit intake of saturated fats and strictly avoid trans fats.

4. Vitamins and Minerals These micronutrients contribute immensely to various body functions. Consuming a balanced, varied diet ensures proper intake. Some key ones include Vitamin A, B, C, D, E, K, calcium, potassium and iron, among others.

5.2. Crafting Your Meal Plan

Every individual's nutritional requirements vary based on parameters like age, sex, weight, activity levels, and overall health. Tailoring meal plans to your needs and preferences can keep you excited and consistent.

A good starting point is the "Plate Method". Picture a plate divided into four quarters. Half of the plate should be filled with colorful veggies, a quarter with protein, and a quarter with a whole grain or high-fiber starch. Add a serving of healthy fat, and voila – a balanced meal!

Work on a meal structure best suited to your lifestyle. Typically, three meals and two snacks work well for most people. Make sure to mix a variety of foods across meals to cover all nutrient categories.

5.3. Shopping Smart

A crucial piece of the nutrition puzzle is shopping smart. With a plethora of food choices available, it's essential to make wise choices.

1. `Buying in Bulk` Grains, legumes, and dried spices are well-suited for bulk buying. The trick is to store correctly to avoid spoilage. Use tight-lid containers and keep in cool, dry places.

2. `Frozen Over Fresh` Frozen fruits and veggies retain nutrient value well and are often cheaper than fresh ones. They also reduce the issue of quick spoilage.

3. `Local Farmers and Markets` Buy local and seasonal. Not only is it helping local farmers, but the produce is also fresher and packed with nutrients.

4. `Labels Matter` Read and understand food labels before buying. Beware of hidden sugars and high sodium content. Remember, the shorter the ingredient list, the better.

5.4. Space-Efficient Storage Ideas

Storage is a primary concern for urban dwellers. Here are some ideas to help optimize your food storage, without compromising on variety or nutrition:

1. `Vertical Storage` Maximize wall space by using vertical storage. Install shelves or hanging spice racks. Magnetic knife racks can free up drawer space.

2. `Under furniture` Under-bed or under-couch storage boxes can be used for non-perishable items.

3. `Furniture as Storage` Items like an ottoman or a coffee table with built-in storage can work brilliantly.

5.5. Cooking Healthy in Small Kitchens

Having lesser space doesn't mean compromising on cooking nutritious meals. One-pot meals like soups, stews, or simple stir-fry dishes are not just space-saving but also pack a nutritional punch. Slow cookers and pressure cookers are handy.

Meal prepping can save a lot of time and ensures you always have healthy options on hand. Make batches for a few days, store correctly, and simply heat and eat!

A nourishing journey needs patience, planning and balance. As you explore and experiment, you fine-tune what works best for you. Remember, this is a flexible blueprint that should adapt to your evolving lifestyle and needs. Adjustment is a part of the game in the pursuit of urban wellness, and learning to do it effectively – that's your ticket to a healthier, happier you.

Make space for fitness, wellness, and particularly, nutrition, even in the smallest of urban dwellings, and watch your life transform!

Chapter 6. Meal Prepping in a Miniature Kitchen

Urban living often goes hand-in-hand with compact kitchens. However, a small kitchen doesn't mean you need to compromise on meal prepping effectively. With the right strategies, tips, and tools, you can still prepare a week's worth of nutritious meals even in the tiniest of kitchens.

6.1. Understanding Your Small Kitchen Space

Before we begin the meal preparation journey, it's essential to get to know your kitchen space better. A comprehensive understanding of your space will help you maximize it effectively.

Start by studying the layout of your kitchen. Identify areas that can be utilized better, such as corners, under cabinets, or even wall spaces that are free. You can use these spaces for storage or setting up necessary kitchen tools.

In tiny kitchens, every square inch counts. Vertically arranged tools, pegboards for hanging items, and magnetic racks for knives and spices can save valuable counter space while keeping your kitchen organized and efficient.

6.2. Essential Kitchen Tools for Effective Meal Prep

Just like larger kitchens, smaller ones need a few essential tools for efficient and effective meal prep. Since space is at a premium, opt for multi-functional kitchen gadgets that can reduce cooking time and save storage space.

1. A Set of Good Quality, Sharp Knives: A chef's knife, a paring knife, and a serrated knife can handle almost all of your kitchen tasks.

2. Food Processor: A mini food processor can be stored easily and takes care of chopping, blending, and mixing.

3. Versatile Cookware: Opt for a high-quality pot and pan that can be used in the oven and on all types of stovetops, including induction.

4. Collapsible Silicone Containers: These are space-saving and ideal for storing prepped fruits, vegetables, and meals.

5. Stackable Mixing Bowls with Lids: These work as mixing bowls, serving bowls, and even storage containers.

6.3. Planning and Organizing Your Meals

Meal prepping is all about planning. By mapping out your meals for the week, you can streamline ingredient use, minimize food waste, and increase efficiency in a small kitchen.

Here are steps you can take to plan your meals:

1. Start by considering your diet, lifestyle, and nutritional needs.

2. Choose recipes that share common ingredients to further simplify meal prep.

3. Write a detailed grocery list based on your chosen recipes to prevent overbuying.

4. Schedule a specific time for meal prepping. Consider a time of the week when you're less likely to be disturbed.

Remember, your meal plan doesn't need to be overly complex. Stick to simple, nourishing, and delicious meals that can be cooked in bulk and are easily reheatable.

6.4. Prepping the Ingredients

Once you have planned your meals and shopped for groceries, it's time to prep your ingredients. Prepping ingredients involve washing, chopping, and sometimes even pre-cooking them to save time throughout the week. In a small kitchen, remaining organized during this stage is critically important.

Try to clean as you go to avoid clutter. Once you're done prepping one ingredient, clean the board, knives, or any other utensils you used before moving on to the next. Piling dishes can be stressful and can take up valuable workspace.

To keep your ingredients fresh, you can use airtight containers or sealable bags. Label your containers with content and the date of preparation to keep track of their freshness.

6.5. Cooking Your Meals

With your ingredients prepped and ready to go, it's time to start cooking. You can choose to cook all your meals at once, or in stages, depending on your schedule and fridge space.

When cooking in a small kitchen, it can be beneficial to adopt one-pot or one-pan recipes. These can drastically minimize the amount of cleaning up and allow you to make the most of your limited stove space.

Prioritize cooking larger batches of flexible base ingredients which can be incorporated into various meals. For example, quinoa can serve as a base for salads, bowls and can even be added to soups.

6.6. Storing Your Meals

Once your meals are ready, they need to be stored correctly to maintain their freshness and ensure ease of use throughout the week. Again, using space-efficient storage methods like stackable containers and collapsible silicone bags is key here.

Store your meals in the fridge or freezer labeled with their contents and the date they were made. If freezing meals, ensure they're properly defrosted before reheating and consuming.

Remember, your freezer is your friend. It can be a lifesaver in a small kitchen, helping you maximize the longevity of your prepped meals and ingredients.

6.7. Boosting Your Meal Prep Experience

Even in a small space, meal prepping can be enjoyable. Create a playlist or an audiobook queue to listen to while you chop and cook. Invest in a set of good quality, durable and sharp tools that make the job easier.

Fully embracing the limits of your tiny kitchen, instead of fighting against them, can lead to unexpectedly creative meals and a rewarding meal prepping experience.

With effective techniques, the right tools, and a can-do mindset, you can transform your miniature kitchen into a powerful ally in your quest for urban wellness. Meal prepping in a small kitchen is not only possible but can also become an enjoyable, fulfilling routine in your journey to a healthier lifestyle.

Chapter 7. Physically Fit, Nutritionally Sound: Balanced Living in the Metropolis

In your bustling metropolitan lifestyle, keeping physically fit and nutritionally sound is crucial to maintain your energy levels and overall wellness. With restricted city spaces, this can be a challenge, but certainly not insurmountable. Welcome to a resourceful guide on streamlining fitness regimes and enhancing nutrition despite small living quarters. This journey will provide you with comprehensive strategies to create a healthful harmony in a fast-paced urban life.

7.1. Urban Fitness: Compact Yet Effective

For city dwellers, finding time and space for exercise can seem like a daunting task. But, not to worry - modern fitness solutions are versatile and adaptable enough even for a 500-square-feet studio. Here is where the concept of compact fitness flows magnificently onto the scene.

NOTE There are three primary ways to approach small-scale fitness: 1. Equipment minimalism 2. Space-utilizing workouts 3. Outdoors turned gymnasium

Equipment Minimalism

The market today proliferates with compact, easy-to-store exercise equipment. Resistance bands, yoga mats, compact dumbbells, and portable pull-up bars are perfect examples. These can be tucked away when not in use, eliminating clutter and ensuring your limited urban dwelling isn't compromised.

A study published in ACSM's Health & Fitness Journal found that High-Intensity Circuit Training (HICT) using body weight as resistance can be an efficient workout. Designed to be completed in a small space, HICT includes exercises like push-ups, burpees, and lunges that can be all conveniently performed within the confines of a small city apartment.

Space-Utilizing Workouts

Workouts such as yoga, Pilates, and martial arts are examples of regimes that require minimal space but offer maximal fitness returns. These exercises not only enhance your strength and flexibility but also relieve stress – a common issue for city dwellers.

Outdoors Turned Gymnasium

You don't need a backyard to enjoy outdoor exercises. City parks, bridges, stairs, or even your apartment rooftop can be transformed into your workout base. With activities like jogging, skiing, bicycling, step climbing, or just brisk walking, the cityscape becomes an urban gymnasium.

7.2. The Nutritious Plate: Eating Smart in the City

Living in a city often means fast food or quick, unhealthy meals due to time crunch. But you can rewrite this narrative. The key to maintaining a healthy diet lies in careful planning, smart grocery shopping, and mindful cooking.

NOTE Here are few strategies to help you eat well in the metropolis: 1. Prepare meal plans 2. Smart grocery

shopping 3. Quick, Nutritious Cooking 4. Cultivate
Healthier Eating Habits

Prepare Meal Plans

Planning your meals can prevent last-minute unhealthy food choices.
At the start of the week, create a menu that incorporates all required
nutrients but doesn't require hours on the stove. With a detailed
meal plan, you can avoid falling into the fast-food trap.

Smart Grocery Shopping

Smart grocery shopping means buying whole, unprocessed foods.
Fresh fruits and vegetables, lean proteins, healthy fats, and whole
grains should top your list. Consider shopping for groceries online to
save commuting time and receive the freshest farm produce.

Quick, Nutritious Cooking

Invest in a slow cooker, rice cooker, or pressure cooker. These
appliances can help you prepare nutritious meals while you're out
working or running errands. You can also use this strategy to prepare
meals in batches to save time.

Cultivate Healthier Eating Habits

Eating healthier is not just about what you eat, but also how you eat.
Include mindful practices such as eating without distractions,
savoring the flavor, and drinking an ample amount of water for
overall good health.

7.3. Wellness Practices: Breathing Life Into Your Urban Existence

Achieving balanced living in a city requires beyond physical fitness
and a well-rounded diet. Here, the concept of wellness comes into

play. Discover the perfect blend of activities designed to enliven your spirit, rejuvenate your mind, and invigorate your body.

NOTE — Here are a few wellness practices ideal for city living: 1. Meditation 2. Deep Breathing 3. Indulge yourself in arts and culture

Meditation

City living can sometimes be stressful and overwhelming. Practicing meditation can help combat stress, promote relaxation, and improve your overall wellbeing. Choose a quiet corner of your apartment for this practice.

Deep Breathing

Something as simple as deep breathing can help lower stress and promote relaxation. It's an incredibly important practice that can be done anytime, anywhere, even amid the skyscrapers!

Indulge in Arts and Culture

City life is often rich in arts and culture. Enjoying these elements can provide a mental health boost. Attend concerts, art festivals, or theatre productions to engage your mind in a positive, enriching environment.

The muscular, spirited metropolis can present challenges when it comes to maintaining a healthy lifestyle. However, armed with the right strategies and an open mind, you can create a wellness oasis right within the beating heart of the city. Always remember, urban living need not equate to unhealthy living. Now, it's time to flex those muscles, eat those greens, and take a deep breath in your very own city sanctuary.

Chapter 8. Turning Limitations into Opportunities: The Mindset Shift

As an urban dweller, the first step to adapting to small-space living is to embrace a mindset shift — seeing limitations not as barriers but as unique opportunities for creativity and innovation. This chapter is dedicated to examining how you can adopt such a mindset, and turn what many perceive as obstacles into your distinct advantages in your journey to urban wellness.

8.1. The Art of Adaptation

Humans are remarkable adapters; it's an intrinsic part of our survival instinct. We have thrived in diverse environments, from vast plains to mountains, and with the rise of civilization, we are adapting even to the concrete jungles of urban landscapes. Similarly, our approach to fitness and wellness needs to be adaptive when faced with the small-space living.

An adaptive mindset towards wellness means being flexible, creative, and resourceful. It means that instead of lamenting the lack of space, we look for total body workouts that can be done on a yoga mat. Instead of feeling constrained by limited kitchen resources, we explore clever nutrition hacks that require minimal ingredients to provide maximal benefits. By seeing the constraints as a challenge rather than a setback, we can create a fitness routine that is uniquely our own.

8.2. Embracing the Minimalist Approach

One of the most effective ways to shift your mindset when it comes to small-space living is to embrace minimalism. Minimalism goes beyond reducing physical clutter; it refers to an overall simplification of your lifestyle. In this context, a minimalist approach encourages the functional utilisation of space, economy in equipment, and simplicity in exercises.

By embracing this approach, you will not just make the most out of your limited space, but also streamline your routine, remove non-essential items, and focus on what's truly helpful for your wellness goals. For instance, using resistance bands instead of an entire set of dumbbells, or practising bodyweight exercises instead of machine workouts, you can convert even the tiniest bedroom corner into your personal gym.

8.3. Seeing Space in New Ways

A critical aspect of turning limitations into opportunities is to change the way you perceive your space.

Look at your small space with a fresh set of eyes, and you will start noticing numerous unexploited potentials. The side of your coffee table could serve as a ballet barre for stretches. Your sturdy dining chair can become your partner for tricep dips or step-ups. The small corridor is perfect for lunges. The entire space, however constrained, can become an arena for high-intensity interval training (HIIT) workouts.

In the kitchen, consider the elevated countertops as your space for cutting vegetables while standing, an excellent subtle workout for your core. Revise your idea of regular lunch by incorporating standing lunches or seated on an exercise ball to promote core stability and correct posture.

8.4. Being Resourceful

Resourcefulness is key when working within constraints. This attitude goes hand in hand with the previously mentioned minimalist approach. In the kitchen, a resourceful mindset could mean learning to prepare nutrient-rich meals using fewer ingredients, mastering the art of one-pot cooking, or finding creative ways to elevate meals with simple garnishes or spices.

Similarly, in the realm of fitness, resourcefulness may imply finding multipurpose use for your yoga mat — yoga, pilates, strength training or meditation; it could serve all. It might mean using household items as workout tools, or learning to substitute traditional gym exercises with equally effective bodyweight exercises.

8.5. Positive Affirmation and Gratitude

Shifting your mindset is not just about practical strategies. It also entails maintaining a positive mental state. Positive affirmations and practising gratitude can be remarkably influential in convincing yourself to view your situation in a new light.

Reframing your thoughts with positivity allows you to embrace your small space, rather than resenting it. Constant gratitude for what you have will instill a sense of contentment and happiness – two important aspects of wellness – into your life.

Conclusively, turning limitations into opportunities in the world of urban wellness necessitates a comprehensive shift in mindset. This shift involves seeing the positive side of constraints, adopting a minimalist approach, innovating space usage, being resourceful, and maintaining a positive attitude along with the practice of gratitude.

This mindset not only allows us to effectively navigate the challenges of small-space living but also equips us to live fulfilling, healthy lives despite any perceived limitations.

Your city space, regardless of its size, can be the starting point of an incredible wellness journey. Every limitation can be converted into an opportunity with creativity, innovation, and a positive outlook. The key is to open your mind to possibilities and to remember — health and wellness are not bound by the size of your space but by the size of your vision and dedication.

Chapter 9. Exploring the Hidden Greenery: Urban Outdoor Fitness

Urban lifestyle, cramped as it may be, brings with it a unique charm and vitality. Among soaring skyscrapers and thrumming roadways, there lie hidden pockets of lush greenery that serve as perfect settings for a phenomenal outdoor workout. Tap into these urban oases. They not only promote physical health but contribute to stress relief, emotional wellbeing, and augment a greater connect with nature.

9.1. The Hidden Workout Oases

When you think city, you see concrete. But let's refocus that lens to find the verdant expanses dotting your urban sprawl. From public parks to waterfronts, pedestrian-friendly streets, and even community gardens, there's an array of spaces within the heart city waiting to be transformed into your outdoor gym.

Keep your eyes open for winding paths ideal for jogging, park benches for step ups, trees for resistance bands, and broad patches of grass for core exercises. You'll realize how an ordinary landscape transforms into an extraordinary fitness routine.

And, don't overlook your own apartment complex! Stairwells make for excellent cardio workouts, terraces for meditative yoga, and even that little corner garden can become a mini high-intensity interval training (HIIT) zone.

9.2. Utilizing City Architecture for Fitness

The city's architecture offers more than aesthetic appeal. It's a potential goldmine for urban fitness enthusiasts. Consider the variety of stairs, railings, walls, ramps, and ledges you encounter daily! Tried and tested urban workouts include stair sprints, ledge pull-ups, wall sits, and ramp sprints.

Exploring these architectural-assets fuses fitness into your regular commute or lunch break walk, making the cityscape an extension of your fitness regime. Choose different spots to workout each day, and you'll never lack novelty or challenge in your fitness routine.

9.3. Adopting Outdoor Sports

Outdoor sports run the gamut from football, cycling, and cricket to more unorthodox fitness options like parkour. With a small group of fitness enthusiasts, any open space can transform into a sporting arena. Not only does this foster camaraderie but also keeps motivation running high.

If group activities aren't your flavor, consider sports like cycling or rollerblading. They offer a unique blend of cardio and strength training and let you cover more ground in your greenery exploration.

Adopting a sport means more than just keeping fit; it's about learning, refining skills, and engaging with your environment in a fun and dynamic way.

9.4. Transformational Green Exercises

Getting in touch with nature can transform your fitness regimen. Here are a few green exercises that you can seamlessly integrate into your daily routine:

- Morning Yoga: A peaceful morning routine that balances your mind and body.

- Tai Chi: A slow, restorative martial art form.

- Jogging: An effective cardio workout.

- High-Intensity Interval Training (HIIT): A full-body workout focusing on quick, intense bursts of exercise.

- Zumba: Dance your way to fitness!

Remember, your work-out space does not limit the intensity of your workout.

9.5. The Power of Group Workouts

Group exercises in open spaces can be incredibly rejuvenating. Boot camps, yoga classes, Zumba events, or even a casual game of football leverage the fresh air and natural surroundings to provide an uplifting atmosphere.

Moreover, group workouts foster a sense of community and accountability. The motivation and encouragement inherent to these settings often lead to more consistent and effective workouts.

9.6. An Urban Fitness Toolkit

An urban outdoor fitness-kit is your trusty companion. This kit is compact and portable, including versatile items like resistance bands, jumping rope, yoga mat, portable kettlebell, and even TRX training kits. Incorporate these tools to further diversify your outdoor workouts.

9.7. The Indispensable Role of Safety

Safety should always be at the forefront of your fitness journey. Ensure that you equip yourself with reflective gear for early morning or evening routines. Stay hydrated, protect your skin with appropriate clothing and sunscreen, and be cognizant of traffic and personal safety in public spaces.

Your ultimate goal is not only about physical prowess but holistic wellness. As urban dwellers, it's time we embraced the verdant pockets of tranquility interspersed amidst our high-rises. Let's convert each corner into a stepping stone towards a fitter, healthier lifestyle. The bustling city can cohabitate with serene wellness if we merely take the time to explore the endless possibilities.

In the upcoming section, we pivot from our outdoor fitness exploration to the vibrant art of in-home workouts within urban spaces. Tight quarters can become large arenas of wellbeing, and we are excited to show you how. Stay tuned.

Chapter 10. The Power of Yoga and Meditation in Limited Spaces

The city hustle often overshadows the importance of a peaceful mind. Yoga and meditation have emerged as potent tools to balance the frantic lifestyle. These practices deliver multiple benefits—physical strength, flexibility, stress reduction, improved focus, and over time, a discernible improvement in the quality of life. The beauty of yoga and meditation is their adaptability. You don't need an expansive yoga studio or a secluded hilltop. You can experience their power right in your compact city living spaces.

10.1. Building a Dedicated Space

Every wellness journey in a small abode starts with crafting a dedicated wellness space. For yoga and meditation, you'll need a spot that accommodates a yoga mat and offers a calm atmosphere. It could be by your bedside, in the living room corner, on a balcony, or beside a window overlooking the cityscape. Equip this space with a yoga mat, a cushion for meditative practices, and maybe few indoor plants for that natural touch. Lighting plays a vital role in creating the perfect ambience. Opt for softer lights, or even better, natural daylight.

10.2. Yoga for the Urban Living

Yoga is an overarching term covering a range of practices from gentle stretches to intense workouts. Here are some yoga practices that cater to the constraints of a limited space.

10.2.1. Sun Salutation (Surya Namaskara)

A simple and compact sequence of poses that warms up your body, enhances flexibility, and encourages mindfulness. You can perform sun salutation regardless of the size of your space.

10.2.2. Standing Poses

A series of standing poses such as Mountain Pose (Tadasana), Warrior Series, or Triangle Pose (Trikonasana) are perfect for limited spaces. They strengthen your muscles, enhance your stability and balance, and they don't require a lot of room.

10.2.3. Seated Poses

Seated poses like Forward Bend (Paschimottanasana), Butterfly Pose (Baddha Konasana), or Seated Twist (Ardha Matsyendrasana) can be done on your mat in a tiny area. They help in toning your muscles, enhancing flexibility, and cultivating inner peace.

10.3. Meditation in Miniature Spaces

Meditation is an inward journey. It's about taming the mind, enhancing focus, and connecting with yourself – tasks you can performed anywhere. Here are some effective meditation techniques for your small city space.

10.3.1. Mindfulness Meditation

To practice mindfulness, choose a quiet space in your home. Sit comfortably, close your eyes, and start to pay attention to your breath. As you breathe in and out, let your mind chatter fade away.

10.3.2. Guided Meditation

Thanks to the digital age, we have access to a plethora of guided meditations. All you need is a device, a pair of headphones, and your chosen spot.

10.3.3. Mantra Meditation

Mantra Meditation or Japa involves repetition of a word or phrase. Mantras can be said aloud or silently. This technique is perfectly adaptable to compact spaces.

10.4. Maintaining Consistency and Discipline

While limited space fitness presents challenges, maintaining consistency and discipline can turn these limitations into a unique wellness terrain. Set up a schedule for your yoga and meditation practices. A daily 30-minute morning session could be a great way to kickstart your day.

10.5. Nurturing a Wellness Community

Living in a bustling city shouldn't isolate you from nurturing a wellness community. Attend local yoga classes or meditation meets. Touch base with like-minded city dwellers and grow mutually.

In sum, the size of your living space needn't limit your journey to wellness. Although invisibly small, the path to inner peace, physical strength and mental well-being is infinitely vast. Yoga and meditation can help you traverse this path, right in the comfort of your small city apartment. Build your practice, be consistent, and the city's chaos will transform into harmony. Embrace your compact living space and let it become a hatchery for holistic health. Harmony isn't a luxury but a necessity. Harness the power of yoga and meditation to shape your urban wellness, one breath at a time.

Chapter 11. Small Space, Big Change: Transformative Fitness Case Studies

Life in urban spaces necessitates creative solutions to reap the benefits of wellness. In this chapter, we journey through a series of transformative fitness case studies that offer invaluable insights on how to make a small space your journey's launch pad towards better health and fitness.

11.1. Meet John: The Homebased Yogi

John, a keen software developer, resides in a 500-square-foot apartment in Downtown Manhattan. Limited space didn't shrink his determination to cultivate a wellness routine. Having always appreciated the serenity of yoga, he repurposed an often underutilized corner of his living room to create a meditative space.

Using a compact, foldable yoga mat and a simple shelving unit to store essential props like blocks, straps, and a bolster, John adheres to a daily 30-minute yoga routine. He finds free online yoga classes to continue refining his poses. His disciplined approach keeps his mind and body nimble, despite the tight square footage.

11.2. Amelia: The Living Room Fitness Enthusiast

Amelia, a marketing consultant from Toronto, has transformed her living room into a versatile fitness arena. She uses apps like Nike Training Club and 7 Minute Workout for variety, and invests in multiuse fitness equipment: A kettlebell for strength training, a resistance band for flexibility, and a stability ball that doubles as her desk chair to improve her posture.

Faced with the challenge of limited storage, Amelia opts for a stylish ottoman that conveniently stores her fitness gear, doubling as a coffee table or additional seating when needed. Her commitment to her workout routine enhances her fitness level, proving that a compact living room can be transformed into an efficient workout zone.

11.3. Grace, Tai Chi and Open Spaces

Grace, a retired professor, lives in a studio apartment in San Francisco. Her commitment to wellness inspired her to devise an adaptable Tai Chi and meditation routine that leverages community parks in her neighborhood.

Her apartment may not have a spacious lawn, but concrete jungles offer several communal green spaces that promote wellness. Her daily routine includes a trip to the local park for Tai Chi exercises supplemented with mindfulness meditation. She emphasizes how the urban dweller can benefit from public spaces to maintain an active lifestyle and build a sense of community.

11.4. Leonardo's Kitchen Gym

Leonardo, a young freelancer in Madrid, exploited the potential of his kitchen to stay fit. With an extendable pull-up bar in the door frame and compact dumbbells tucked away in the cupboard, his kitchen is his temple of fitness.

Leonardo augments his routine with exercises utilising furniture: tricep dips on the chair, inclined push-ups against the counter, or step-ups on a sturdy stool. This ingenious use of household items asserts that the journey to health requires determination, not enormous spaces.

11.5. Emma's Balcony Garden

Emma, living in a high-rise in London, found solace in balcony gardening. While gardening isn't a conventional workout, it provides dynamic stretching, squatting, and lifting movements that aid in maintaining her flexibility and strength.

Her compact garden offers fresh, nutritious produce, and she makes it a point to share excess produce with her neighbours. It's not just her physical health that benefits from her hobby - sharing her produce fosters an invaluable sense of community.

Every space holds potential. These individuals, each residing in different corners of the urban world, represent the tenacity of the human spirit, proving that wellness can be achieved even within the confines of small, urban dwellings. The journey to wellness isn't about how much space you have, but how you utilize it.